What peop

CW00347453

"I have known Colin   at
time, he has demonstn   .al
wellbeing, health and fitness. Throughout that time, he has
maintained a desire to retain his excellent good health and
general wellbeing by researching many products and ideas
before discovering the genuine health benefits of bee
propolis. Since then he has become an acknowledged expert
in his field.

I am sure you will enjoy reading the book and, by taking his
advice and guidance, enjoy the many benefits of bee
propolis."

– Dr Neil Lancaster, DBA, MSC, BA (Hons) FCIPD.

"I first met Colin in 1956 when we were in our late teens.
We had many shared interests, one of which was motor
cycling.

We had great adventures on our bikes, the most memorable
was that of pass storming in Europe on my 650cc Triumph
Thunderbird. He was a devoted to keep fit enthusiast and
still is, having run a marathon in his 60s and many half
marathons.

Open water swimming in his 70s and scuba diving were
other pastimes he enjoyed. Colin is very dedicated in
anything he does, and I wish him all the best in his future
endeavors."

– John A.Vauvelle.

Praise for bee propolis listed in Healing Help from Honeybees

"I have been using bee propolis for more than 11 years now, and colds and flu have become distant memories. I always take two capsules a week or so before a holiday flight, to keep the cabin bugs at bay. It works."

– *Percival: Immune System Booster.*

"Taking these tablets has helped my hay fever massively. It used to be seasonally debilitating with streaming eyes and a sore nose. I usually take propolis a good week or two before the season gets established. I swear by this bee product, and constantly recommend it to my family and friends."

– *Berry: Boost for hay fever*

Healing Help from Honeybees

How bee propolis can heal burns, wounds, acne, eczema and more

Colin Platt

Contents

Acknowledgments

Writing a book about my passion for the World of Bees would not have been easy without the help of family and friends. In particular I would like to thank my wife Judy who has helped, not especially with the writing, but with encouragement to persevere to completion.

Thank you to my son and daughter Anthony (Tony) and Pippa for their love and support and for never doubting my ability to finish my book.

Thank you to Cathy Brockhill for word processing help. Without her, this book would have taken much longer to come to fruition.

To Manda Waller for her enthusiastic proofreading and copy-editing contribution.

Finally, I would like to thank Christopher John Payne who has written more than 20 books of his own and been involved with close to 200 books for clients and others. He helped me significantly with this book, and his son Toby helped with the formatting.

About the Author

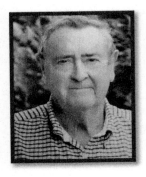

Colin is an acknowledged expert in the medicinal properties and value of bee propolis, following many years of personal use.

Now in his 80s, he attributes his vibrant health and vitality to this magical substance. He has written this book to show the astonishing impact propolis can have on longevity, quality of life, and long-term health for you and your family.

Save the Bees

Rather than ignore the catastrophic decline of our bee population I have added a brief comment on page 75 to the fact that we should all be aware of our bee predicament, and that we all have to contribute in keeping our environment clean and free from pesticides and man-made pollution. But nonetheless, a short section on the miracle of bees.

Bees are involved in the processes for much of global food production and perform about 80% of pollination worldwide.

In recent years, bee colonies have been disappearing at a rate that is alarming for our farmers, whether growing grains, fruit, nuts or flowers.

The use of pesticides has been blamed. But there are many other factors involved, such as man-made pollutants and the destruction of our Rain forests and Fauna.

Many are now establishing new hives in our cities, in small spaces on balconies, gardens, and green spaces. At least it's a start.

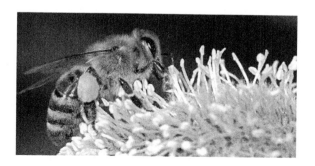

Introduction

The flu season was once again with us. A different seasonal flu virus had been forecast for this particular winter. Hospitals were preparing for more admissions than normal. Hopefully, the new vaccine would help to ease the situation.

My bouts of colds and flu were becoming more regular and so intense that they had become emergency situations. There is a sense of a switch being flicked when you struggle to breathe and begin to realize that oxygen is the source of human life which we all take for granted. We can live without food for many weeks, water for just a few days, but oxygen for just a few minutes.

"If you've ever experienced the agony of flu symptoms, a distressing cold or a chronic cough, when you feel that your lungs are on fire, you'll know that it can be a terrifying experience as you struggle to breathe".

Finally, I came down with a chest infection so serious I found myself in a hospital bed, on a ventilator, struggling to breathe. The effects of these serious chest infections can turn your life into threatening events, and no way did I wish to experience another traumatic episode.

It became a mission—an obsession if you like—firstly to never personally suffer these effects again, and then to help others to overcome this common, unpleasant ailment.

remedies which seemed to ease the symptoms, such as garlic, ginger, Echinacea, and vitamin C. But what was needed was a supplement to **prevent** life threatening episodes.

Maybe an exercise regime could help? As someone who smokes a pack of cigarettes most days, I was aware that I was doing myself no favors. I knew I had to stop this dangerous habit and start a serious fitness regime...but what?

I had always been keen on sport, but participation had taken a back seat as the responsibilities of daily family life and work projects took priority.

Unexpectedly, I had some good fortune. It was Christmas and a family member gave me a best-selling book by Jim Fixx. Published in 1977, *The Complete Book of Running* is an amazing, inspiring book. Jim Fixx is credited with helping start America's fitness revolution, popularizing the sport of running and demonstrating the health benefits of regular jogging. This was just the sort of inspiration I needed to kick start my fitness regime.

It's strange how coincidences happen just at the right time for me, and this was one of them. Another one was to follow very shortly when I discovered the healing help from honeybees.

Just months after reading Jim's book, I had become an enthusiastic jogger and was enjoying my running regime at a local club. As luck would have it, the club had some spare tickets for the Boston Marathon. This is the oldest public marathon in the world. When it started in April 1897, just 15 runners elected to run the 32.2 miles course. Today, 30,000 is the limit.

As with all life-changing events, I distinctly remember the circumstances in great detail.

It was a cold, frosty morning in January 2006 and, in preparation for the Boston Marathon, five of us had arranged a training session. One of the runners in our group, a pilot captain from a major airline, talked about how his hay fever and asthma used to impact on his ability to train. He told us how a friend had recommended he try a natural bee product to help his hay fever and asthma.

Since then, some seven years had passed, and he had never suffered from these ailments again. As a bonus, he'd had no colds or flu either!

He talked about these supplements constantly and enthusiastically during our training runs. Several of his colleagues at the airline had followed his recommendations and had started taking the supplements too — resulting in fewer coughs and sneezes on their flights. This is all the more remarkable as aircraft are well known for being the breeding ground for many common ailments.

When I saw my running friend the following week, he handed me an old well-worn copy of a book by F.Murat published in 1982 titled *The Eternal Natural Healer*. Now out of print, the book covers the many protective properties and immunity boosting benefits of receiving healing help from honey bees.

Apparently, their healing qualities had been known in ancient times and now, slowly, the world was remembering the remarkable properties of this anti-viral powerhouse. Many scientific studies have shown that they could help in treating a vast range of medical conditions, and provide a new frontier for magical healing.

Could this be my Everest?

Now at last there could be a safe natural way to combat these agonising symptoms. An antiviral product, lost for centuries, a powerful natural antibiotic to assist your own body's healing power naturally and boost your immune system.

You may be asking what this book could do for you. Well, dear reader, Healing Help from Honeybees is what you need to read if you care about your health.

Slowly, the world is rediscovering the amazing anti-viral properties of bee propolis and its ability to increase the production of antibodies in the human body, and over the course of this book I will show you just how powerful it can be.

In the field of nutritional medicine our first line of defence is **prevention rather than cure.** Instead of waiting for infections to start and then using drugs from the pharmacy to kill the infectious bacteria we should adopt the ancient Chinese methods and strive to keep well rather than the reverse.

Modern research has shown that as propolis was found to be effective in many ways such as...

- A strengthened immune system.

- A protection against the flu virus.

- Prevents re-occurring respiratory problems.

- An effective remedy to combat bronchitis.

- A natural antibiotic alternative.

Even the ancient Greeks, recognised how powerful propolis was, with Hippocrates (460-337 BC) reputed to be the 'father' of modern medicine recognising its antibacterial properties.

This eternal natural healer has been proven to not only to suppress colds and flu but to alleviate Sinus infections.

It is also a fact that the true cost to Industry and Commerce in terms of lost workdays, production costs and profits is almost incalculable, plus the personal cost in lost income and social activity.

Now, for just a few cents per day you can save on these expensive Physician's visits and over the counter cures.

More than one third of patients who saw a doctor received an antibiotic prescription which adds up to 41 million prescriptions in the USA alone according to the World Health Organisation at a cost of $1 billion.

In the USA the common cold leads to 75 to 100 million Physician visits per annum at a conservative cost of $7.5 billion, and in over the counter drugs Americans spend $2.9 billion and another $400 million on prescriptions for symptom relief.

Annually this of course has a massive implication for antibiotic resistance.

This constant overuse has contributed to mutations of bacteria into resistant strains turning simple infections into serious life-threatening illnesses, over which we have less and less control. Doctor George Jacoby of the Harvard Medical School does not beat about the bush when he states that "Bugs are always figuring a way around the antibiotics we throw at them then they come roaring back." It would appear that bugs and bacteria are cleverer than man.

For a fraction of the cost I had found a remedy which didn't need antibiotics.

Here is a sample of what you will learn inside:

- How to say goodbye to harmful antibiotics.

- How to fight your colds and flu the right way.

- How to save upwards of $997 a year on medical bills.

- How to treat your children safely too.

- How this natural antibiotic can alleviate throat infections.

- How propolis relieves halitosis (bad breath) and gum disorders.

The Flu

Although often confused with the common cold, flu is a more severe condition, causing a fever and muscle pains along with a sore throat and coughing. The symptoms last for days, or even longer.

Imagine **never having to seriously suffer** again from one of these agonising symptoms. According to the World Health Organisation, tens of millions of people contract seasonal flu every year. It can be fatal, some patients—mostly the elderly and the very young—can die.

Even healthy people can be affected, and at any age. In particular, people over the age of 50, very young children and those who have chronic medical conditions are more likely to get complications such as pneumonia, sinusitis, bronchitis and painful ear infections.

So why take chances with your health? With your family's health?

It's good to know what you are up against. So, a brief explanation of the type 'A' virus (which causes the most severe illness) is interesting. It can be subdivided into different types.

- H1N1. Caused Spanish flu in 1918/1920. Truly a global pandemic spreading even to the Arctic, killing 40 to 100 million people. 99% of deaths occurred in people under 65 years old, and more than half of the deaths were in young adults in the 20 to 40 age bracket. This pandemic has been described as "THE greatest medical holocaust in history and may have killed as many people as the Black Death". **Swine flu falls into this category**. Could this be the next pandemic? This type of flu can be passed from person to person, simply by human contact, or via contaminated surfaces, such as door handles, elevator buttons and public places.

19

- H2N2. Known as ASIAN flu in 1957-1958. Killed 1 to 1.5 million people.

- H3N2. Known as HONG KONG flu killed 0.75 to 1 million people.

- H5N1 or AVIAN flu or bird flu as it is known, is the latest Pandemic threat 2008-2009. Due now, and known as the **"Coming Plague"** it is being taken very seriously indeed by responsible governments particularly by the USA, UK and Europe. Flu jabs are being stockpiled in their millions in anticipation of the immediate threat, but production is limited. Demand will massively exceed supply. So, who will be selected, who will be prioritised?

The last place you want to go in the event of a pandemic is hospital. They will be totally unprepared in a major event.

But we can help ourselves. Those with the knowledge of this natural preventative have proved its effectiveness time and time again.

Protection and prevention is in our hands **now**. It is y**our** responsibility to protect yourself and keep yourself healthy, as no one else will...

So, You Have Two Choices

Either: Be pro-active for yourself and your family, and discover the remarkable medicinal properties of this 'gift' from nature. Keep these dangerous ailments at bay with this proven natural bee remedy. The truth is, you cannot afford to take any more risks with your health, especially with increasingly resistant cold and flu strains on the horizon.

Or: Continue to be plagued by all these illnesses, and expensive physician's bills. Don't forget the spectre of a 'superbug' (H5N1 avian flu) resistant to all known antibiotics is rapidly approaching, and it will be the **'Survival of the Fittest'.**

As I have already described, I was tired of spending year after year on the miserable merry-go-round of contagious illness, battling the coughs, congestion, sore throats, sinus infections, body aches and fatigue of colds and flu. I searched for a remedy until I found it: propolis. Since then, I haven't had a cold, or flu, or any other contagious illness for many years.

Now I want to pass that miracle remedy on to you.

Many people can't believe there's one miracle substance found in nature that possesses the key to fighting infection. This substance not only kills pathogens, but strengthens the body's immune system. Modern scientific research has found it to be the only substance in the world that's been proven to be antibiotic, anti-bacterial, anti-fungal AND anti-viral, all at the same time. An amazing by-product from bees that's been used for over 3,000 years.

This miracle substance is PROPOLIS. In reading this book, you'll learn everything you need to know about propolis, from its creation by bees, to its use by the ancient Egyptians and Greeks, to the ways it can prevent and treat myriad illnesses.

You will also learn about the new super-bugs that have learned to outsmart antibiotics, but have been scientifically proven to be vanquished by propolis.

Some people think the chances of a natural substance like propolis successfully fighting antibiotic-resistant bacteria and killer viruses is about as likely as winning an Iron Man event when you can't even swim.

Read on and you will have a new understanding of this miracle substance from the hive.

I have not written this book for the sole purpose of converting you from using orthodox allopathic medicine. Instead, I want to open your eyes to a natural product that, although not in its infancy, is a substance that you may know little about. A substance that could be truly a benefit to you in its use.

May this information bring you health, happiness and the miracles of healing.

1

The Defender of the Hive

Everybody knows that bees make honey, but few know the crucial part that propolis plays in the life cycle of the Western Honeybee (Apis Mellifera). **The fact is, without propolis, there would fewer bees, no hives and no honey...**

What is propolis?

Propolis (also known as bee glue or bee putty) is a mixture of tree resin and bee secretions used in the construction and maintenance of beehives. Just as bees gather pollen and nectar to bring back to the hive for food, they collect plant resins to make propolis.

"It's no wonder the adage "Busy as a bee" was coined. Honeybees have been known to travel up to 12 square miles on pollen and resin gathering missions."

In northern regions, the resins come primarily from poplar, pine and balsam trees. In southern climes, bees gather resins from certain flowers, as well as trees. After mixing it with a combination of saliva and beeswax, they stash the mixture in their storage sacs for the journey back to the hive.

Chemical analysis reveals that propolis is a complex amalgam of plant resin, beeswax, aromatic oils and bee pollen. Its hue varies from golden brown to almost black, with occasional green or red tints. Naturally, the color and the exact makeup of propolis varies according to the botanical source of the resin and the area of the bee's habitat.

Propolis is to bees what penicillin is to various forms of bacteria, or at least, what penicillin *was* before bacteria learned to outsmart it. But the difference is we don't encase our homes in penicillin to ensure that they stay disease-free. Bees, those clever little engineers, *do* seal their homes with propolis to keep it **sterile.**

Because as many as 40,000 bees are apt to live in a single hive, it's imperative that the warm, dark, humid environment be kept free of mold, fungus and disease. And what bees have figured out in the 125 million years that they've been buzzing around the Earth, is that propolis is the most powerful antibacterial substance found in nature.

Bees use the sticky substance to line their walls and stop up cracks when they construct their hives. Virtually every surface in the hive is coated with a thin layer of the sterilizing substance. They also encase the hive entrance with a narrow tunnel of propolis. In order to get in and out of the hive, the bees must crawl through the tunnel, which cleanses them of dangerous bacteria and keeps the hive safe for its inhabitants. If by chance a spider, or some other foreign body enters the hive that's too big to be carried out by the bees, they swathe it in a thick cocoon of propolis, in effect mummifying it to ensure that it doesn't contaminate their home with mold or fungus.

Another clever use of propolis prevents one of the honeybee's natural enemies from making a mass assault on their hive. Ants like honey (not to mention larvae and dead bees) as much, or more, than humans, and will go to great lengths to swarm into a hive en masse, kill the inhabitants and consume the delicious amber syrup within. Bees have devised an ingenious strategy to foil ant attacks using, you guessed it, propolis. Painting a thick layer of the sticky resin at the hive's entrance, the bees immobilize the ants long enough to sting them to death and thwart their attack.

Bees also spread a thin blanket of propolis over the cells of their honeycomb, keeping it bacteria free. This is crucial for the survival of the species, because honeycomb holds the hive's most important treasures (aside from the queen), bee larvae, pollen and honey.

Propolis also serves to reinforce the honeycomb, adding to its tensile strength. Perhaps this is why honeycomb, which is made primarily of wax, is able to hold loads of up to 25 times its weight in honey.

2

A History of Propolis

It is believed that primitive humans enjoyed the fruits of the industrious little honey bee, dining on royal jelly, honey, honeycomb and larvae. However, it was the ancient Greeks who gave propolis the name we use today. *Pro* means *before,* and *polis* refers to *city*. Thus, *'before the city'* acknowledges that bees line the entrance of the hive with propolis, keeping it safe from infection and intruders. Some say that a more apt translation is, *'in defense of the city'*. And propolis truly is the defender of the city of bees, the hive.

About 3,000 years before the Greeks used propolis; the Egyptians employed it in one of their most sacred rites; mummification. In order to preserve their dead and guarantee an auspicious afterlife, they melted down the whole beehive—honey, honeycomb, propolis, wax and all. Strips of linen were soaked in the mixture and wrapped around the body, forming an effective preservative cocoon to limit fungus, mold and decomposition.

Propolis was the primary ingredient of prized incense used in ancient Greece. Mixed with aromatic herbs and burned on charcoal, it emitted a delicate, but sublime perfume.

The Greeks, as well as the Egyptians, Sumerians and Babylonians also immersed their dead in vats of honey, which served as a remarkably effective preservative. Alexander the Great is among several notable Greeks who received a honey immersion burial.

The philosopher and scholar Aristotle (around 350 BC) was the first to undertake detailed research on the antiseptic and healing properties of propolis. He built a glass hive to better observe honeybee workings, but the bees, preferring to conduct their business in darkness, promptly coated the glass in propolis. Despite the bee's desire to obscure their nest, Aristotle gleaned significant insight into their realm and made noteworthy advances in the knowledge of their industry. He chronicled the antiseptic quality of propolis and recommended its use for a variety of ailments, including bruises and sprains.

Hippocrates, holder of the illustrious title, "Father of Modern Medicine", prescribed propolis for sores and ulcers. The Greeks were the first known civilization to promote beekeeping as an endeavor worthy of cultivation. The healthful properties of bee products became so well known throughout Greece, that they boasted as many as 20,000 cultivated hives by the year 400 BC.

In Rome, Pliny the Elder (23–79 AD) further advanced the knowledge of propolis in his treatise *Natural History*, identifying three distinct types of the substance. He noted that propolis was commonly prescribed by physicians to reduce swelling, extract material embedded in the flesh, and heal wounds that were so severe as to have been deemed incurable.

References have been found in the Koran to the medicinal properties of honey and propolis, confirming that the ancient Arabic world was also in tune with apiarian remedies.

Eastern European medical journals from the 13th century document the use of propolis to relieve tooth decay. It's also known to have been used as a remedy for inflammations, abscesses, canker sores and respiratory infections.

Because of its anti-bacterial and anti-fungal properties, propolis was used to treat wounds during the Boer War in South Africa in the late 1800s.

It was dubbed 'Russian penicillin' in World War II, when the Soviet military used it as wound dressing. A piece of propolis slowly dissolved in the mouth is an age-old sore throat and canker sore remedy recommended by beekeepers. Propolis lozenges are sold all over the world to heal and soothe a sore throat. Although bee-product remedies were largely discarded in the West in favor of synthetic pharmaceuticals in the latter part of the 20th Century, their resurgence is burgeoning, particularly as modern antibiotics are proving increasingly ineffective against mutating strains of viruses and bacteria.

Healthcare providers are seeking new ways of staving off potentially catastrophic epidemics which modern pharmaceuticals are unable to treat. Could it be that a centuries-old product from the hive will re-emerge as the magic bullet they've been looking for?

3

Super-bugs, a worldwide threat

Today's headlines are full of alarming news about so-called 'super-bugs' that are immune to modern pharmaceutical treatment. Epidemiologists are increasingly concerned about these new, rapidly mutating viruses and antibiotic-resistant bacteria that have the potential to infect billions of people. The potential for a worldwide pandemic is enormous.

A review of some of the findings:

In the United States, the Journal of the American Medical Association reported that over 94,000 people were infected with antibiotic-resistant

Twenty-five million pounds of antibiotics, or 70% of all the antibiotics produced are fed to livestock in the U.S. each year. Because of repeated exposure to antibiotics, pathogens have morphed into more resistant strains in order to survive.

staphylococcus in 2005. Of those 94,000 people, 18,650, or roughly 20%, died of the infection. In Europe, studies show that streptococcus pneumonia has become resistant to penicillin almost 50% of the time. Other reports reveal that large numbers of soldiers returning from Afghanistan and Iraq have contracted wound infections that are resistant to antibiotics. Flesh-eating bacteria (necrotizing fasciitis) are also cause for concern. A little over a year ago, a woman in the U.S. had almost half of her upper body (hand, arm, shoulder and breast) sequentially amputated after she was attacked by the infection, which is caused by an antibiotic-resistant form of strep A. She was fortunate—the disease usually kills its victims within 72 hours.

Avian or bird flu is first known to have morphed from chickens to humans in 1997. Because of its resistance to all known anti-viral medications, experts believe the H5N1 virus has the ability to become a worldwide pandemic, killing billions of people. It had a 50% mortality rate when it spread throughout Asia in 2003 and has since cropped up in Africa, Europe and the Middle East, causing the deaths of over 200 people and killing an estimated hundreds of millions of birds. Currently the virus is only known to have the ability to be passed from infected birds to humans, but epidemiologists fear that it may have discovered a way to be transmitted from human to human. (See more on this subject in Chapter 7.)

Although health experts thought that modern antibiotics had relegated tuberculosis to the dustbin of medical history, they've recently had cause to reconsider. A new, virtually untreatable form of tuberculosis (XDR-TB) is impervious to antibiotics. The strain has cropped up in India, causing alarmingly high mortality rates. The World Health Organization fears that XDR-TB is set to become a deadly global health threat. These kinds of outbreaks have prompted the U.S. Center for Disease Control to state that antibiotic-resistant bacteria is one of the world's most pressing problems, adding that, "Over the last decade, almost every type of bacteria has become stronger and less responsive to antibiotic treatment."

Researchers believe that the reason for this is twofold: First, the widespread overuse of antibiotics by the general public. Since penicillin was invented in the 1940s, people have learned to rely on antibiotics to an extreme degree. Doctors, often at the patient's insistence, will prescribe antibiotics at the drop of a hat, even for maladies like viral infections on which they have no remedial effect whatsoever.

Secondly, the use of antibiotics in livestock: Although the use of antibiotics as a preventative treatment in the commercial livestock industry has been largely banned throughout the EU, the U.S. still employs the practice, pumping huge quantities of the drugs into animal feed. In industrial style livestock production, antibiotics ameliorate the negative health effects of overcrowding and unsanitary conditions.

Bacteria have survived on the earth longer than man or beast. In fact, bacteria were the first forms of life on earth and have been around for four billion years. Like all living things, they have their own innate intelligence and ability to evolve in a way that guarantees their survival.

Bees, it seems, have found a way to beat bacteria at the survival game with a miraculous substance created from plant resins. If we want to protect ourselves from constantly evolving pathogens, we can take a lesson from the bees and turn to propolis to safeguard our health.

4

The Good News: A Miracle Antibiotic from the Hive

As you learned in earlier chapters, propolis possesses a phenomenal array of curative properties, including anti-fungal, antibacterial, anti-inflammatory, antibiotic, antacid and anti-tumor.

It is used to treat a wide spectrum of health problems: arthritis, muscle soreness, respiratory illness, prostate inflammation, skin disorders, chronic fatigue syndrome, burns, tooth decay, allergies, herpes, endometriosis, menstrual cramps, Candida, infertility, wounds, urinary tract infections, ulcers, laryngitis, parasites, smallpox, canker sores, tumors and digestive disorders.

How many times have you come in contact with a fellow worker who thinks they're doing everyone a favor by coming to work with a cold or flu? This walking Petri dish, sniffling, sneezing, coughing and generally infecting everyone around them, will no longer be cause for alarm if you're fortifying your defenses with propolis!

Many people, including myself, now take propolis regularly for general health maintenance, finding that it strengthens their immune system and decreases the incidence of colds, bronchial infections and flu.

With a fortified immune system, we can keep ourselves healthy in even the most virus and germ infected environments. There are many testimonials from people who used to get colds and flu every year. Since taking propolis, they've breezed through cold and flu season with nary a sneeze, ache, sore throat or sniffle. Medical researchers, for whom modern synthetic drugs were once a Holy Grail, have tried to determine why propolis is able to treat such a vast number of disorders.

They attempted to isolate the various chemical properties of propolis in hopes of finding one active component that's responsible for its effects. Because it has more than 150 chemical properties and because those chemical components depend on the botanical source, propolis is difficult to analyze. Nevertheless, researchers have found that no one component is responsible for the curative effects of propolis.

In fact, when the chemical components of propolis are isolated, they don't work effectively. Rather, propolis combines all of its properties to create a synergistic effect. In simple terms, it's the sum of its parts, rather than any one component that enables this miracle from nature's pharmacy to do its curative work.

Another property of propolis is that, unlike synthetic antibiotics, it doesn't destroy the good bacteria with the bad. Anyone who's taken antibiotics and has then come down with a yeast infection, an upset stomach, or diarrhea, knows that synthetic antibiotics are undiscriminating in their war on bacteria. Because our bodies maintain a complex system of bacterial equilibrium in order to stay healthy, destroying bacteria indiscriminately creates its own set of problems. This is another reason why propolis is so special.

We might use this analogy in describing propolis use: If our bodies were a castle in danger of being invaded by an army of enemy marauders, it would make more sense to reinforce the wall surrounding the castle, rather than to set off a bomb which would indiscriminately destroy the wall and the marauders alike. Propolis has also been shown to work in conjunction with synthetic antibiotics.

Studies in Brazil, Australia and Bulgaria show that propolis boosts the effectiveness of penicillin and other antibiotics by as much as 100 %. Another study using propolis in conjunction with amoxicillin, ampicillin and cefalexin in fighting salmonella showed a synergistic effect in increasing efficacy. Propolis also reduces the amount of synthetic antibiotics administered to patients, thus reducing the side effects. What are the chemical compounds of this miracle healer? 40% to 50% of propolis is made up of resins, which are rich in flavonoids.

To sum it up: propolis is one of the most powerful natural healing agents known to man. It has the ability to disarm a wide variety of pathogens and cure a vast array of illnesses.

Flavonoids exist in all blossoming plants, but they have different properties when found in propolis. Experts believe that the enzymes excreted in bee saliva when the bees process propolis produce a chemical change in the flavonoids. There are many different types of flavonoids, but the most important ones found in propolis are pinocembrin and galangin, which have significant therapeutic properties. Flavonoids are shown to strengthen the protein shell surrounding viruses which renders the virus harmless.

Propolis has phenolic compounds, including caffeic acid phenethyl ester, which has been shown to inhibit the growth of cancer cells and reduce inflammation.

Flavonoids comprise as much as 20% of the biochemical properties of propolis, which might explain why it's such powerful natural healing agent.

Flavonoids exist in all blossoming plants, but they have different properties when found in propolis. Experts believe that the enzymes excreted in bee saliva when the bees process propolis produce a chemical change in the flavonoids. There are many different types of flavonoids, but the most important ones found in propolis are pinocembrin and galangin, which have significant therapeutic properties. Flavonoids are shown to strengthen the protein shell surrounding viruses which renders the virus harmless.

Propolis has phenolic compounds, including caffeic acid phenethyl ester, which has been shown to inhibit the growth of cancer cells and reduce inflammation.

Propolis also contains essential minerals and trace elements such as calcium, magnesium, copper, potassium, manganese, phosphorus, iron, cobalt, silica and zinc. Perhaps most importantly, propolis can be taken regularly as a preventative, health-boosting measure, ensuring good health and vitality and keeping illness at bay, no matter what the circumstance.

It's important to note that propolis may cause an allergic reaction in some people. You should take the necessary precautions when you begin using propolis, by taking only very small quantities at first. Once you determine that you don't have an allergy to it, you can begin taking a full dose.

You are more likely to be allergic to propolis if:

- You have a severe allergy to bee stings.

- You are allergic to bee pollen or honey.

- You are allergic to evergreens, poplar or balsam trees.

- You have asthma.

You should also avoid using propolis if you are pregnant or nursing, just as you would take precaution when using any form of medication. **Do not stop using prescribed medication without consulting a professional medical practitioner.**

5

Scientific Studies on Propolis

As worldwide health organizations recognize that modern pharmaceuticals are becoming ineffective in combating illness-causing bacteria and viruses; they begin to look for alternative treatments. But the fact is, scientific research on the health effects of propolis has been going on for over sixty years.

Western research on propolis began in the 1960s in Denmark and France with studies by Dr. Remy Chauvin and Dr. Aagard Lund. Dr. Chauvin, who conducted his research at the Sorbonne in Paris, is considered the world's foremost authority on propolis. Dr. Aagard developed a process of cleaning and preserving propolis that is still

Chauvin also points out that propolis bestows significant amounts of vitamins and minerals when taken internally, while antibiotics do the opposite, causing deficiencies in these important nutrients.

considered state-of-the-art today. Chauvin states, "Scientists believe that nature has a cure for every disease. It's just a matter of finding it. With the introduction of propolis, it is possible that we can one day abolish most drug-related chemicals. Also, remember that keeping the body free from diseases through natural healing can actually slow down the aging process and add years to the lifespan." The antibacterial and anti-viral properties of propolis work to raise the body's natural resistance to disease by internally stimulating one's own immune system. Since Chauvin began to tout the miracle healing powers of propolis, scientific studies on the subject have risen dramatically, with over 300 scientific studies conducted on propolis between 1980 and 2010, and these numbers are increasing.

These studies verify what the ancients learned centuries ago: propolis is truly a miracle healer, capable of eradicating both viruses and bacterial infections, something no other substance is known to do.

Some of the recent research conducted on propolis:

- Researchers at the University of Western Australia have found that propolis can increase the effectiveness of penicillin or other antibiotics anywhere from 10 to 100 times. Studies done in Bulgaria and Brazil corroborate these findings.

- Research by Dr. Ali F. M. at the Ain Shams University in Egypt found that propolis successfully treats infertility associated with mild endometriosis with virtually no side effects.

- Research done at the Department of Microbiology, University of Alabama at Birmingham confirmed the existence of anti-microbial agents in various bee products, using streptococci bacteria as a test.

- A study at the Instituto de Ciências Biomédicas da Universidade de São Paulo, Brazil and the Graduate

Institute of Food Science and Technology at National Taiwan University, both concluded that propolis inhibits the growth of staphylococcus aureus.

- The Department of Science at the Università degli Studi di Roma La Sapienza, Roma, Italy studied ethanolic extract of propolis in conjunction with antibacterial drugs on staphylococcus aureus. The scientists concluded: "Our results indicated that the extract of propolis had a significant anti-microbial activity towards all tested clinical strains. Adding the extract to antibacterial tested drugs, it drastically increased the anti-microbial effect of ampicillin, gentamycin and streptomycin, moderately the one of chloramphenicol, ceftriaxon and vancomycin, while there was no effect with erithromycin. Moreover, our results pointed out an inhibitory action of the extract on lipase activity of 18 staphylococcus spp. strains and an inhibitory effect on coagulate of 11 s. aureus tested strains."

- The Department of Microbiology and Immunology, Silesian Academy of Medicine, Zabrze-Rokitnica, Poland concluded: "Ethanolic extract of propolis exerts a strong anti-bacterial activity, in addition to anti-fungal, anti-viral and anti-protozoa properties. In previous studies at these laboratories we have demonstrated that the intensity of the bactericidal activity of the extract is correlated with the virulence of the mycobacterium tested, and that this extract has a synergistic effect with antibiotics on growth of staphylococcus aurous."

- The Department of Biochemistry, University of Oxford, United Kingdom conducted research too:

"The effect of the natural bee product propolis on the physiology of microorganisms was investigated using B. subtilis, E. coli and R. spheroids. An ethanol extract of propolis had a bactericidal effect caused by the presence of very active ingredients. The exact bactericidal effect of propolis was species dependent: it was effective against gram-positive and some gram-negative bacteria."

- The Departamento de Microbiologia, Laboratório de Biologia de Microrganismos in Brazil conducted a study of propolis ethanol extract for inhibitory activity against mouth ulcers. Their results stated, "All of the assayed bacteria were destroyed by propolis extract".

- The Department of Oral Biology, Faculty of Dentistry, Hebrew University-Hadassah, in Jerusalem, Israel conducted the following study: "To investigate the antibacterial properties of propolis and honey against oral bacteria in vitro [in an artificial environment] and in vivo [in a living organism.]" RESULTS: Propolis demonstrated an antibacterial effect both in vitro on isolated oral streptococci and in the clinical study on salivary bacterial counts.

6

Forms of Propolis

Because of increased awareness of the vast array of healing properties of propolis, it is now available in a variety of forms and can be purchased at most health food stores and many pharmacies.

Propolis preservation was first researched by Dr. Aagard Lund, mentioned in Chapter 5 for his propolis work in the 1960s and 1970s. Lund was the first to develop a process for preserving propolis. His process is still used by many producers today to ensure the integrity of propolis' healing properties.

Just as you would with any product, it is important to get propolis from a reputable source. Because propolis is extremely sticky, it absorbs pollutants from the air. Therefore, it's important to gather propolis from an organic clean area.

After propolis is gathered and cleaned of extraneous material, the active components are extracted by soaking it in alcohol. Then the mixture is dehydrated, either using a vacuum process, a spray process or a freezing process, at which time a wide variety of propolis products are produced, such as:

- Capsules: These are available in two forms, either liquid propolis encased in capsules; or powdered propolis, encased in capsules. Both are taken orally for a variety of ailments.

- Tinctures: Propolis in a base of water, alcohol or propylene glycol. Can be taken internally or externally, though it can stain the skin if applied externally.

- Lozenges: Propolis extract prepared with honey or sugar. Used for sore throats and coughs.

- Throat spray: Good sore throat soother.

- Nasal spray: Used for inflamed and clogged sinus passages. Both nasal and throat aerosols can be used for halitosis (bad breath) or mouth sores. Can also be used externally for cuts, rashes and fungal infections.

- Cough syrup: Soothes a sore throat and inflamed bronchial tissues, thus quieting a cough.

- Creams: Usually a 2% liquid propolis solution mixed in a cream base. Used for skin problems such as eczema, dermatitis, psoriasis and burns. Also used as an anti-aging cream because of its ability to improve skin elasticity.

- Ointments: Same preparation as with the cream, but the propolis is mixed in an oil base. Used for the same conditions as cream.

- Shampoo: Propolis extract added to shampoo formula. Used to invigorate and nourish the scalp and hair. Can stain hair, so it needs to be a low propolis concentration.

- Soap: Especially good for acne treatment and other skin conditions.

- Toothpaste: Good preventative for gum disease and halitosis.

- Gum: Believed to help dental hygiene and halitosis.

- Lip balm: Used to treat chapped lips and cold sores.

A list of conditions and treatment options with propolis:

- Acne: Propolis cream, ointment, capsule or tincture.

- Burns: Propolis cream, ointment, tincture, lip balm.

- Dermatitis: Propolis cream, ointment, tincture, lip balm.

- Eczema: Propolis cream, ointment, lip balm.

- Gum problems: Propolis capsule, tincture, toothpaste, chewing gum.

- Health Maintenance: Propolis capsule, tincture.

- Herpes: Propolis cream, ointment, tincture, lip balm.

- Laryngitis: Propolis capsule, tincture, cough syrup.

- Sore throat: Propolis capsule, tincture, cough syrup.

- Yeast infections: Propolis cream, capsule, ointment, tincture.

Despite the plethora of packaged propolis products, it's believed that the best way to administer it is to chew the pure form taken directly from the hive. Care should be exercised if taking scrapings from the floor of the hive as they might contain debris and impurities.

The visible impurities are most likely to be small slivers of timber or wood from the hive, as the bees make sure that there is a good seal to cover any cracks and ingress of water.

If the beekeeper does not attend the hive regularly then the propolis can harden and more force has to be used, sometimes causing cosmetic damage to the hive.

Again, use propolis in tiny quantities until you determine that you don't have an allergy to it. The allergy can be in the form of itchiness of the skin, maybe a rash and skin irritation. Do not use if you have a bee allergy, or if you are pregnant or nursing.

Do not stop using prescribed medication without consulting a professional medical practitioner.

7

A Global Health Crisis in the Making: Avian Flu

Unfortunately, just because avian influenza (also known as bird flu or H5N1 virus) has all but disappeared from the headlines, doesn't mean we can rest easy. Avian flu is currently one of the deadliest viruses in the world, with the potential to kill billions of people. There is currently no known way of controlling the spread of avian flu. No one will be immune to it.

In March of 2008, the United Nations Food and Agriculture Organization (FAO) issued a warning that the risk of an avian flu mutating into a human pandemic form is growing increasingly possible.

In Indonesia and Egypt, the virus appears to have mutated into a new strain, rendering attempts to develop a vaccine useless.

The chief veterinary officer of the UN's FAO says that unless the disease is contained at its source in animals, there will be many more cases of transmission to humans. Currently the virus can only be passed from birds to humans, but the more human cases of H5N1, the more likely it is that the virus will learn how to migrate from human-to-human. Once it evolves into a form that can be transmitted within the human species, a worldwide epidemic of historic proportions will likely follow.

There are two methods by which H5N1 can improve its ability to be transmitted among humans. The first is what scientists call a 'reassortment event', whereby human and avian viruses exchange genetic material. This would occur during simultaneous infection of a human or a pig. In this case, the virus would obtain the ability to infect humans, exploding into a worldwide pandemic.

The virus can be transmitted by touching contaminated surfaces. Anyone who comes in contact with someone with the virus runs the risk of contracting it.

The second method of evolution happens when the virus gradually develops the ability to bind to human cells. This involves small clusters of human avian influenza infections, with some incidence of human-to-human transmission. According to some accounts, this may already be occurring.

The first known human outbreak of avian influenza linked directly to chickens was in Hong Kong in 1997. Since then, the virus has spread throughout Asia, also making its route through Egypt, Turkey and Romania.

Indonesia is the biggest source of avian influenza, with an estimated 30 million people continuing to raise chickens in close proximity to humans, despite the health risk. Indonesia has reported 129 cases of the virus to date. Of those known cases, 105, or 81%, were fatal.

H5N1 is highly contagious from poultry contact. Anyone working with poultry, eating undercooked poultry, or traveling in a country affected by the virus is at increased risk for contracting avian flu. The movement of H5N1 virus into wild bird populations further increases the risk of an epidemic. A survey in the EU found 741 cases of avian flu in wild birds between February and May of 2006. The birds were identified in the UK, France, Greece, Italy, Hungary, Slovenia, Germany, Austria, Slovakia, Sweden and Poland.

Most of the infected wild birds have been swans, but ducks, geese and birds of prey have also been found to carry the virus. The good news: propolis, with its ability to kill virus pathogens, may be the best bet when it comes to protecting ourselves against avian flu. At this point, no scientific studies have been done to determine propolis' effect on the H5N1 virus. However, it's quite possible that the most powerful anti-viral, anti-bacterial, anti-fungal substance found in nature will also prove effective in fighting avian flu.

No other substance has the ability to boost the immune system and eliminate pathogens. Propolis could very well divert a devastating avian influenza pandemic, which currently has no other means of remedy.

More H5N1 facts (from The World Health Organization):

- Domestic ducks now appear to be silent bearers of avian flu, having developed the ability to infect other birds without exhibiting symptoms of the illness. They excrete large amounts of the virus in their feces, further increasing the risk of spreading the disease. Because they do not appear to be sick, humans and other birds are more likely to come in contact with infected ducks, thus increasing transmission of the virus.

- Researchers have compared the H5N1 viruses from 1997 and 2004, and found that they've become more deadly and are able to survive longer in the environment.

- Avian flu has widened its host range. It now infects and kills mammals that were previously considered resistant to infection with the virus. An unprecedented die-off of wild birds occurred in China in 2005, when more than 6,000 migratory birds were killed by avian flu.

- The 1918 flu pandemic killed an estimated 40 million people. An avian flu epidemic is expected to have a much higher mortality rate.

- Because of the large numbers of people requiring medical treatment, health services will be overwhelmed by an avian flu pandemic. High rates of health worker infection will further hamper attempts to treat the sick.

- Other essential services, such as transportation, communications, governmental and law enforcement agencies will be negatively impacted in their ability to function, due to worker infection.

- The ability of international relief organizations to offer assistance during a pandemic will likely be suspended, due to the need to contain the spread of the virus by limiting travel.

- Because the H5N1 virus is constantly mutating, vaccines are not expected to become available until several months after the start of an epidemic. Current vaccine production capacity falls far short of the amount needed to treat a pandemic.

- There are currently only two drugs known to treat influenza, oseltamivir (Tamiflu) and zanamivi (Relenza). Both must be administered within 48 hours of the onset of symptoms. There is no clinical proof that these drugs are effective against the H5N1 virus.

At current manufacturing capacity, it will take at least 10 years to produce enough of the above-mentioned drugs to treat just 20% of the world's population. The bottom line, propolis, the miracle remedy from the hive, could help stave off a killer flu pandemic in two ways:

1) It strengthens the immune system, enabling the body to use its own infection-fighting defenses more effectively and...

2) By its ability to kill deadly pathogens, including viruses, on contact.

Avian flu or bird flu (H5N1) is a very serious threat. The World Health Organization (W.H.O.) fears that avian flu could kill millions in the next few years given the high volume of global traffic.

Most large cities and towns already have contingency plans in place to deal with the problem.

8

Conditions Helped by Propolis

The Russians have probably done the most research in discovering the antibiotic, anti-inflammatory, and antibacterial properties of propolis in 1947 at the Kazan Veterinary Institute, so much so that propolis came to be known as 'Russian penicillin', prior to this date, it was being used and applied to slow healing wounds during the Boer War, and again during the Second World War in Russia.

Reports in the use of this amazing substance have become legendary. When Dr. Bernard Jenson Ph.D. visited the Caucasus people in Russia, he found that, "All the oldest men in the area had been beekeepers and used raw honey AND hive scrapings as a regular part of their diet." He interviewed one of the beekeepers Shirali Mislimov who was 157 years old!

Coughs and Colds

In 1989 Polish researchers gauged the effects of propolis on groups with the common cold. The group treated with propolis had the infection for a shorter period, with complete recovery within 3 days. The untreated group took five days to recover. Research into its uses showed that it is more effective as a

prophylactic i.e. preventing catching the ailment rather than curing it. The old adage 'prevention is better than cure' rings true!

Researchers have found that the best results seem to be obtained by taking 1 to 1.5 grams per day, but do recommend backing off for a week every three months to prevent the body becoming over sensitized

Influenza and Flu

We all know that flu is a viral infection and that as a rule, antibiotics are not medically prescribed, as they are of little value, except in cases of a severe respiratory infection. I have found, and other propolis users have also confirmed that one is less likely to catch flu, but if you do suffer it is not as severe.

In May 1976 a particular virulent Flu epidemic swept through the town of Sarajevo. Professor Izet Osmanagic a local resident conducted a trial and chose a control group who were in particular danger of becoming exposed to the epidemic, namely, student nurses and teachers.

Each was instructed to take propolis and honey every day for a certain period.

Sixty-five nurses and teachers who were without symptoms took the product and 157 did not. Only about one in ten of the students who took propolis were infected and out of the 157 in the control group, one in four contracted the epidemic. The teachers faired even better as only one in twenty-five had a mild attack.

Dr. Kravcuk of Kiev found that propolis was effective against sore throats and dry coughs in 90% of two hundred and sixty cases. Dr. Remy Chauvin of Paris, France concurs. "Propolis works by raising the body's natural resistance to infection; through stimulating one's own immune system.

Dosage to Help: To stay well up to 2000mg daily, in capsule or tablet form.

Although I have researched and used propolis extensively, during my studies of the subject I have come across a wide range of benefits attributed to this amazing natural product, ranging from Acne to Ulcers!

Let me table for you, some of the wide-ranging results, as confirmed by a world authority James Fearnley of the UK.

In James Fernley's LLB book "Bee Propolis" 2001, he tables user's experiences with propolis as follows:

	Positive	Negative	Too Soon
Arthritis and muscular pain	89%	7%	4%
General health maintenance	89%	0%	11%
Respiratory problems	76%	7%	17%
Skin problems	90%	9%	1%

Chronic fatigue syndrome	63%	16%	21%
Stomach and digestive disorders	69%	9%	22%

The important survey of users using propolis was well received and exceeded all expectations. The 'Too Soon' column relates to those who were yet to see results. Notice the efficacy of skin problems and how quickly their conditions improved.

Acne and skin problems

It can be seen from the table above that skin problems scored a 90% positive result in the use of propolis. Many people have reported suffering with Acne for years and applying propolis cream has shown its effectiveness within just a few weeks.

A tincture of propolis can be used but it can have a temporary staining effect on the skin.

Doctor Edith Lauder of Vienna in her clinic used propolis tinctures and creams on more than twenty cases of *acne simplex* which were completely healed by home application within a week.

Her most memorable result was in the treating of a woman who had been treated unsuccessfully for thirty years with *acne conglobata* on her face and chin. The condition was cleared after just a few visits to her clinic. She had many more notable successes in treating dermatology conditions.

Dosage to help: Use propolis cream and tinctures. (Tinctures can stain the skin). Propolis soap is now available, and. its use can be recommended for acne treatment.

Arthritis

The above table is a positive indication of the effectiveness of propolis. Many people are unable to take anti-inflammatory medication due mainly to the adverse effect it has on the lining of the stomach and have turned to this more natural product.

A poultice consisting of least 10% propolis and beeswax has been found to be beneficial, the propolis absorbed by the skin works as an anti-inflammatory, analgesic and the heat is said to increase joint mobility by improving blood circulation in the area affected.

Dosage to help: Daily up to 2000mg of propolis capsules or tablets.

Alzheimer's

It was reported as far back in March 1998 of an extraordinary event with propolis given to an elderly patient by Sister Carole of the Little Sisters of the Poor to alleviate a recurring chest infection which was not responding to antibiotics. Within days the chest problem was resolved, but the propolis treatment triggered a positive side effect on the patient who had symptoms of Alzheimer's. She appeared more alert and had a more of an interest in her surroundings and other patients.

Sister Carole continued to give propolis to a further twelve patients at St. Josephs Home in Newcastle, England, and ten more patients in Lambeth London all suffering from the same condition. All showed a marked improvement to their quality of life. The improvement in the patients' condition was gradual and positive.

"I'm not claiming to have found a magic cure, but the results have been extraordinary", says Sister Carole. Don't you love stories with a happy ending?

Asthma

If you do not have an allergy to honey or bee stings, then Asthma could be treated effectively with propolis by inhibiting the inflammatory process present in respiratory ailments.

Since taking propolis, an Asthma sufferer for many years felt as though he had 'new lungs.'

Dosage to Help: Daily up to 2000mg daily. Tincture of propolis is a more concentrated form and can have a more immediate effect to stave the onset of an asthma attack.

Many people take 500 mg per day. I take double this dose, simply to stay well and keep my immune system in trim.

Authorities recommend a break every 6 or 8 weeks for a week at a time.

Bronchitis

Honeycomb capping's which contain raw honey and pollen (a higher antibacterial value than pasteurized - none heated - honey which lacks important enzymes) and propolis inhalations was used to treat patients with this condition in Russia. The group was split up 56/48. The former were treated conventionally, the latter with the cappings.

Those taking the honey and propolis inhalations were cured up to 4 days earlier than those treated conventionally with fewer relapses.

Dosage to Help: In the absence of honeycomb cappings, an alternative could be Manuka honey, produced by bees pollinating the Manuka tree in New Zealand.

According to research and the latest studies at Waikato University Research Unit by Professor Molan, are showing that this honey with a UMF® value (Unique Manuka Factor) with a minimum standard of 10 gives an increased antiseptic and antibacterial properties, stimulating the body's immune system and helping the body to deal with infection.

Cancer

As previously mentioned, cancer in beekeepers can be rare. A survey of thousands of beekeeping societies in Germany found that 1 in 3,000 reported having cancer, as opposed to the US where 1 in 4 persons will have cancer in their lifetime. This could be for a variety of reasons. The use of their own pure honey cappings which contains propolis, pollen, and even exposure to sting venom may have something to do with beekeepers' resistance to cancer.

It has also been reported that treatment with a high factor Manuka honey be taken on an empty stomach and 3000mgs capsules daily can ease the cancer treatment.

Chronic Fatigue Syndrome

An ME (Myalgic Encephalomyelitis) survey, sent privately to James Fearnley of Beevital, published the results of 58 of their members in 1997. All Aged between 26 and 67 and having been diagnosed with ME for between 11 months and 14 years.

Of the participants 12 were bedridden or housebound whist nearly one third were very poorly.

They took between 1-12 grams of propolis per day in tablet, tinctures and tablet form.

Out of the 58, 53 reported that taking propolis had made an improvement to their condition almost immediately; one reported an adverse effect and 4 patients were not aware of any change.

Out of 22 people who said that they had reduced or stopped their treatment, 18 reported deterioration, with an immediate improvement once they had restarted treatment.

The effective suggested dosage by the author was about 3000 mg per day, but the more seriously affected patients found relief at between 8-12 g per day.

Patients reported greater mobility, an increase in energy, and a reduction in infections.

Coughs and Colds

A propolis spray has been found to be affective also; propolis and lemon soothers (lozenges) are now available. A persistent cough can be helped by gargling with a propolis tincture mixture 4 or 5 drops taken diluted in a glass of warm water.

The best results can be obtained by taking 1000 to 2000mgs of propolis per day.

Cuts

A non-alcoholic tincture can be applied this will sting less, because of is antibacterial properties it will reduce the risk of infection and effect quicker healing.

Cystitis

Urinary tract infection, an inflammation of the bladder, usually affects women, but can affect either sex or age groups. It is usually treated with antibiotics. Taking two 2000mg capsules daily has been found to be a good alternative, and then one capsule a day long term dosage as a prophylactic (to keep the symptom at bay)

Dental Treatments

The use of propolis in dentistry has become the most popular areas of clinical research in the world and has been the traditional treatment for hundreds of years.

More recently, a German researcher Dr.Schmidt in 1980 conducted a double blind clinical trial of a propolis mouth rinse. The study showed patients with gingivitis (gum inflammation) improved significantly with this method of treatment. Three years later Romanian researchers confirmed the trials of Dr.Schmidt, with propolis and Royal Jelly.

In 1990 a Russian study with propolis confirmed its potency in root canal fillings because of the anesthetic effect and bone generating properties.

Another study in 1991 carried out in Japan on rats found that those given a propolis/water solution, showed less dental deterioration than untreated rats.

Recent studies in the UK have been carried out effectively, thanks to the work by Dr. Philip Wander, a retired cosmetic dentist.

The patients of Dr. Wander who ran several dental practices in the Manchester area of the UK can thank their lucky stars that he has become a worldwide authority in the use of propolis for a wide range of dental problems.

Dr. Wander, amongst his many qualifications gained his Diploma from the Faculty of Homeopathy in 1994 in London, England, specialises in natural dental techniques that minimise discomfort and improve oral health. He advocates the use of propolis mouthwash or gargle for temporary relief of sore throats and gums and halitosis (bad breath).

As long ago as 1995 he reports the experiences of a growing number of his colleagues who are using propolis and tincture to treat painful oral ulcerations, dental trauma and root canal therapy.

He states that propolis has a slight anaesthetic effect as tinctures can be applied to ulcerated areas with a cotton wool bud where other preparations are not so effective at staying in place. Treatment can then be continued by the patient at home.

Another application where he has achieved success is in treating gum inflammation of erupting wisdom teeth. The beauty of this treatment is that pain is relief is immediate much to the relief of grateful patients.

His 'paper' in January 2005 "Health from the Hive, Applications of Propolis in Dentistry" highlights the growing problem of tongue and lip ulcers aggravated by body piercing. His photographs in this article illustrate the before and after effect of tincture application which provides a physical resin barrier and showed significant healing three days later.

His other much publicised paper "Taking the Sting out of Dentistry" (very apt!) mentions other dental applications of propolis tincture such as accelerated healing of extraction sockets, denture stomatitis (inflammation of the gums which can form under dentures...thrush), mouth ulcers, cold sores, and treating dental decay, particularly in children's teeth.

Dr. Wander is the only dental surgeon (up to this date) to have received a fellowship in Dental Homeopathy FFHom from the Faculty of Homeopathy in London. In 2009 he was voted the

8th most influential dentist in the UK in a poll in the publication "Dentistry".

He has written numerous articles promoting dental homeopathy and holistic dentistry, and **now** advises other practitioners on a consultancy basis.

Eczema

Propolis cream can have an amazing effect on dry Eczema. Just apply daily together with up to 2000mgs daily capsules at the start, for a few days.

The Daily Mirror in their Health Extra November 7th, 1994 column reported on the case of their 2-year-old with chronic Eczema. "His skin was red raw, and we hadn't had a proper night's sleep for two years" said his father. "But were amazed at the results when we bought a jar of propolis cream – we could see the difference the next morning".

Endometriosis

A tissue similar to the lining of the uterus which is found elsewhere in the body causing infertility, painful periods and pelvic pain)

A paper presented to the 59th annual meeting of the American Society of Reproductive Medicine in 2003, by Dr. F.M. Ali of the Ain Shams University in Egypt, researched the results of 40 female patients for more than two years.

These patients were given 500mg of propolis twice daily or a placebo for six months. The study showed that among those given the propolis, 60% became pregnant as opposed to 20% given the placebo.

There were no side effects recorded and the trial concluded that bee propolis could be an effective treatment for infertility and mild endometriosis.

Halitosis

Dr. Maximillian Kern, Ljubljana Clinic in Yugoslavia treated halitosis with propolis. Their symptoms entirely disappeared within a few days. After 8 weeks he checked all the patients again and found no reoccurrence of the problem. Regular brushing with propolis toothpaste can help the condition.

Hay Fever

Sufferers have reported a reduction in their symptoms after taking propolis, but it can largely depend on the allergy to a particular type of pollen.

Some people have found relief by taking a spoonful of local honey or local bee pollen a month or so before the start of the pollen season.

Dr Remy Chauvin treated a number of patients in 1980 with a propolis extract for seven days, eight doses daily of 250 mg of propolis extract. The patient's symptoms were completely alleviated in most patients.

Dosage to Help: As above in capsule form.

Laryngitis

The treatment of sore throats, tonsillitis and acute laryngitis has found favor with the use of propolis. Positive effects have been very noticeable.

Researchers in Rumania in 1975 treated over 200 patients with propolis. Ten percent of each group was treated by conventional methods. Those treated with propolis recovered more quickly than the control group.

Dosage to Help: Gargle with a solution of propolis tincture in warm water. The solution can be swallowed for added effect.

Throat lozenges are commercially available and can be used on a daily basis as a booster.

Prostate Problems

Many men after a certain age notice that urinating and flow deteriorates. When it does start it is weak and spasmodic

These symptoms are caused by benign prostatic hyperplasia (BPH), the herbal extract saw palmetto is quite often recommended, particularly in Germany. However, propolis had been clinically tried in 1997 in Bulgaria by Mladenov on 55 patients aged between 55 and 95. All had been recommended for conventional surgery. Honey, propolis, bee pollen and royal jelly were given to patients as individual needs were assessed. After treatment 95 per cent of patients over a period of 8 weeks no longer complained of pain and their prostates returned to normal size.

Shingles

Treatment with propolis has proved effective for this annoying complaint in both capsule form and propolis cream. Two-gram capsule taken daily, and the cream has the effect of eradicating the itching.

Toothaches

Using tincture of propolis on a cotton bud or similar in region of the aching tooth area. This can reduce the pain because of the anesthetic effect of propolis until dental treatment can be affected.

Ulcers

Dr. Franz K. Feiks at the public hospital in Klostereuberg in Austria was one of the first to use propolis to treat stomach ulcers in 1978.

In a clinical study involving 294 patients he found that 90 per cent of 108 patients given a 5 percent extract of propolis 3 times daily were free of symptoms and pain after 2 weeks, compared with only 55 per cent of those conventionally treated. Dr. Feiks found that 70 percent obtained some relief in 3 days.

Propolis is now known to inhibit the growth of MRSA which as we all know is a serious problem in hospitals.

Maybe it will become the answer to this common infection!

I have mentioned Manuka honey from New Zealand previously in this book. A high UMF® (Unique Manuka Factor) value is recommended for oral use, the greater this value the more effective the treatment. This product is usually available from good health food stores.

Warts

Warts are benign growths of the skin caused by a virus and can cause pain and discomfort if not treated.

Dosage to help: A topical application of propolis, at least 50% tincture in alcohol solution applied twice a day for two weeks has proved to be effective.

Wounds

The ancient Egyptians and Greeks over 4000 years ago recognized the healing properties of raw honey applied to burns and wounds, boils and slow healing sores and abscesses.

When the healing processes of modern antibiotics have stopped working the medical profession has turned to honey products.

Contrary to popular belief, one of the best ways to heal a wound is to keep it moist. Now, dressings are available which are made from a highly absorbent material saturated in a high-grade Manuka honey from New Zealand which the experts say kills bacteria and speeds up the healing process.

Clinical trials show that Comvita Medihoney™ eradicates MRSA from venous ulcers.

Treatment to help: Also tincture of propolis should be used owing to its antibacterial properties, and to reduce the risk of infection.

9

Colony Collapse Disorder

The phenomenon of colony collapse occurs when most of the worker bees in a bee colony disappear and leave behind the queen, a few nurse bees, and plenty of food for the remaining immature bees.

Since 1869 the global bee population has suffered a gradual decline. The bee pandemic known as Colony Collapse Disease (CCD) or Mary Celeste Syndrome has erased 50% or more of the bee population.

Honey is in short supply as bee workers desert their queens and once-thriving bee farms are seriously at risk of collapse.

Early in October 2006 in Crawford County, Larry Curtis lost more than 80% of his 1,200 bee colonies in six weeks. By mid-November he had lost 1,000 hives and 100.000lbs of honey.

One of Pennsylvania's biggest commercial beekeepers, Dave Hackenberg of Union County, Lewisburg, found that in mid - November he suddenly lost 50% of the 2,700 colonies he owns. His commercial enterprise pollinates the blueberries in Maine, and oranges in Florida.

The pollination industry in the USA was once a $45 billion industry, but no more. Seasonally hives are transported from state to state, to pollinate the big Californian almond crop and fruit farms in Florida.

"If the bee disappeared off the surface of the globe then man would only have four years of life left" – Albert Einstein

Some say the Varroa mite is the culprit, others pesticides, others mobile phones, GM crops, it is still a mystery.

Bees are the lifeblood of the universe and now beekeepers worldwide are demanding that their respective governments should provide adequate funds to solve the bee pandemic.

There have been demonstrations in Spain and France to draw attention to the need for funds to research CCD and other bee parasites.

On November 5th 2008, thousands of British beekeepers demonstrated in front of No.10 Downing Street, UK, each carrying their hive smokers and placards demanding more action to fix the honey bee problem. As a direct result of this activity, the UK Government has allocated £10 million to research our pollinators including the bees.

But let's face it, we have been exploiting bees since the beginning of time, stealing their honey, desecrating our planet and killing them off without thought or favor. Let us instead respect them, and nurture their habitats.

The problem is not a new event. Bees have been disappearing since the first known event in the USA in 1869. Long before

GM crops were introduced and before pesticides were used. In the UK in the early 1900's 90% of the bee population in the Isle of Wight UK were mysteriously wiped out.

So, this is not a new problem and I hope that the bees with our help can find their own solution.

10

Pollen

Pollen is the male seed of flowers and is produced by the stamen so that the plant can reproduce. The number of stamens in most flowers is the same as the number of petals.

The main function of the stamen is to produce the pollen grains which house the male sex cells necessary for reproduction. Pollen grains vary in size, shape and color.

It is the job of worker bees to collect pollen and deliver it back to the hive. The worker bees are all female but do not have the same abilities as the queen bee. Worker bees are all born sterile. Their purpose is to work for the good of the hive community. This is their lot in life (a woman's work is never done!) and they have a life span of about 45 days. The queen bee, on the other hand, can live for up to 5 years.

The male bees, called drones, are larger than the worker bees. They do no work whatsoever. They have no sting and their job is to service the queen bee to produce up to 2500 eggs per day.

If you have ever studied a worker bee on a flower, you will have noticed it can be overloaded with the pollen that it carries in special sacks on its back legs.

An average worker bee will collect pollen from as many as 1200-1500 flowers from a distance of up to twelve square miles. The pollen grains can vary in color depending on the types of flower visited by the bee. Bee pollen is a mixture of pollen, saliva and nectar or honey and is carried back to the hives and stored in the honeycombs where it ferments and is the bee-food for the whole colony.

A Complete Food

Bee pollen contains many of the nutrients required by the human body. It is well-known by experts as a perfect nutrient-rich source of vitamins and minerals, flavonoids and carotenoids. It is also antibacterial and is similar in many ways to propolis. It also has a high proportion of vitamin B12, which is essential for the formation of oxygen carrying red blood cells and maintaining our nervous system and energy sources.

When bee pollen is given to anemic patients, their levels of hemoglobin increases significantly.

Bee Pollen in your Diet

Bees normally carry more pollen than the colony needs, so beekeepers use special screens to scrape and collect the pollen residue as the bees enter the hive. The tiny brown or orange granules can be eaten directly, made into pollen bars, eaten in capsule or tablet forms, or ground into a powder to sprinkle onto any food including your favorite cereals, smoothies, or yogurt.

The taste of the granules varies depending upon the species of flower visited by the bees.

Interestingly Royden Brown of the C.C.Pollen Company of Scottsdale, Arizona produced a pollen bar for President Ronald Reagan called the "The Presidents Lunch" in honor of the President.

During his years in the White House the President was known to keep a case or two of pollen bars available at all times, which he gave generously to friends and visiting statesmen

The Power of Pollen

The British Olympic Coach Tom McNab was awarded the British Coach of the year in 1972. As one of the world's leaders in sport he has coached international athletes including England's silver winning Rugby Union squad in the 1992 World Cup and also the British Olympic Bobsleigh Team. He was asked to test the effectiveness of bee pollen on athletes under his supervision and found that within 12 months the performances of his squad of athletes had improved substantially.

The Ethiopian runner Abebe Bikila was a life-long user of bee pollen and won an Olympic Gold Medal in 1960 and 1964.

World heavyweight champion Mohammed Ali used bee pollen as a supplement to give him strength and staying power to help him outbox Leon Spinks (a younger opponent) to win the championship for a third time at the age of 36.

Antii Lananaki, coach of the Finnish tracks team had 36 runners under his supervision and revealed that most of his runners took pollen supplements with only positive results. The Finns had 36 runners in the top 100 Olympic runners in the 1972 Olympics, certainly a record year compared to other years.

Alex Woodly the director of the well-known Education Athletic Club in Philadelphia, quotes,

"Bee pollen works and it works perfectly. Pollen allows super-stars to increase their strength and stamina by up to 25%. This increase in strength and endurance may be the key to the secret regenerative power of pollen. Bee pollen causes a definite decrease in pulse rate. The whole beauty of bee pollen is that it's as natural as you can get. No steroids and no chemicals"

Bee pollen has been used in certain cultures for thousands of years but has become increasingly popular in modern times following testimonials from athletes that supplementation increases speed and stamina.

It is also known that bee pollen had been used by American Indians to provide instant energy for their long migrations, and was often carried in a pouch that was worn as a necklace.

Bee Pollen Benefits for Men

A common condition for men over 55 years is an enlargement of the prostate called prostatitis or BPH (Benign Prostatic Hyperplasia) causing it to swell and squeeze the urethra (the urine pipe), making the passing of urine slow and difficult and sometimes very uncomfortable.

A well-known survey was carried out by Swedish doctors who treated over 100 men who had BPH with pollen tablets. It was found that about three quarters of those trialed obtained relief from this condition.

A similar study in Japan was carried out but this time a control group was given a placebo (identical lookalike imitations) instead of bee pollen. Those taking the real pollen in the group showed an improvement in urination of 89% whilst those taking the fake placebo showed no improvement whatsoever.

Bee Pollen Benefits for Women

Studies have shown that a regular use of bee pollen helps to reduce the frequency and intensity of hot flushes and to reduce the menopausal effects of the monthly cycle.

The Federal Ministry of Health in Germany recognizes bee pollen as a medicine and the German health magazine *Naturheilpraxis* in a clinical reported test that bee pollen lowered the risk of heart disease by lowering the blood levels of cholesterol and triglycerides.

As far as cancer is concerned, many medical studies have been carried out and the conclusion is that cancer remission has been reported in cases in which bee pollen had been administered.

Dr.Peter Hernuss from the Vienna University found the above to be the case with a double blind test with 25 women with uterine cancer using chemotherapy. Some were given bee pollen, and some a placebo. Those being treated with pollen showed a distinct increase in cancer antibodies as a result of increase in their red blood cells, and their hair loss was less noticeable with fewer effects of the radiation.

Those women in the placebo control group showed no signs of improvement whatsoever.

11

Honey... Liquid Gold

Honey is one of the most amazing natural products known to man, and in its raw state (untreated) it contains both pollen and propolis. It has been used for 3,000 years as both food and for its healing properties.

When we say raw honey, we mean honey harvested directly from the honey comb by spinning the comb centrifugally and collecting the amber liquid in a suitable container.

It is preferred in its 'raw' state, both for its medicinal use and for human consumption, as it contains both pollen and propolis. The honey we buy in jars has been pasteurized by heating. This reduces its healing properties by removing active enzymes and vitamins such as vitamin C.

Importantly, the antioxidant and anti-microbial effects of honey has been generally accepted as **greater** in the darker colored honey when compared with lighter colored honey.

Manuka Honey

I can go no further without talking in more detail about the famous Manuka Honey from New Zealand, and also a similar honey from Australia that has the same antimicrobial and antiseptic properties.

Nicknamed "Liquid Gold", manuka honey is produced by bees foraging amongst the wild manuka tree shrubs and jelly bush trees which grow predominately in New Zealand and Australia.

The Australian honey is cultivated in undisclosed locations in northern New South Wales, and southeast Queensland. It is made by bees visiting the **jelly bush tree**, or the lemon-scented tea tree.

Researchers testing honey made from this tree in a range of areas in Australia found that some had 1750mg/kg of the antibacterial compound MGO, the highest concentration yet found in this kind of honey. In fact, this is higher than that found in the famous New Zealand manuka honey.

The word manuka though is the Maori word for the tree or bush. The dark fragrant honey is monofloral or unifloral meaning from a single floral source, and famous for its medicinal uses. It stands head and shoulders above other honey types, due to its levels of hydrogen peroxide; a naturally occurring antibiotic found in this honey.

Also, Methylgloxal (MGO) is found in large quantities in manuka honey. This is another powerful antibiotic molecule, which exists in higher concentrations in manuka than in any other honey varieties.

The renowned researcher Dr. Peter Molan from the University of Waikato, (a region of the upper north-western region of New Zealand/Hamilton), published many articles confirming the amazing antibacterial properties of the honey from the manuka tree (Leptospermum Scoparium), a cousin to the myrtle tree.

Dr. Molan confirmed what had been discovered decades earlier—that manuka honey quickly heals infections that are unresponsive to normal antibiotics and antiseptics. It is particularly effective in combatting dangerous penicillin-resistant strains of Staphylococcus.

Oil extracted from the manuka tree (Leptospermum Scoparium) has long been used topically by the Maoris as a salve to cure and prevent bacterial infections such as dermatitis and psoriasis.

Manuka Honey Components

As mentioned above, it is the Methylglyoxal (MGO) compound found in manuka honey which sets it apart from other honeys, as it does not break down when heated and therefore retains more of its antibacterial qualities. These qualities are quantified and graded with a **UMF score** (Unique Manuka Factor) by certain laboratories in New Zealand. The UMF relates to the antibacterial strength and the amount of MGO. The higher the score, the purer and more effective is the honey against bacterial infections, and also the more expensive!

As mentioned previously, the Australian equivalent has higher levels of MGO. Its healing powers and popularity could lead to litigation as to which country has the legal rights to monopolize the trademark "Manuka", resulting in a bitter row between the two countries.

Australian producers are claiming that New Zealand has no exclusivity to claim a monopoly on manuka honey!

Because of its powerful antibiotic properties and its effectiveness for wound treatment, manuka honey has been approved by the U.S. Food and Drug Administration (FDA) in the use of bandages and band aids. It is *hygroscopic*, so when applied to wounds it draws out moisture and pus just like a sponge soaking up water, thus helping to remove harmful bacteria.

Honey is particularly useful in the treatment of sore throats and mouth ulcers (and as previously mentioned, a tincture of propolis as used by Dr. Wander in his dental practice the UK was found to be just as effective in treating gum infections as conventional antibiotics with less risk.)

Novak Djokovic the ace tennis player in his autobiography has endorsed manuka honey as a key part of the organic diet that helped to revive his career when he was discovered to be gluten intolerant.

Another fan of this 'liquid gold' is Kourtney Kardashian who uses manuka as a face mask, and feeds the honey to her children to ward off colds and flu.

Healing with Honey

Manuka honey dressings are made up from a light viscose mesh with 100% medical grade manuka honey.

According to Dr. Molan, the honey has been used to heal many types of wounds and chronic skin infections successfully. In studies of 600 patients, no adverse reactions were evident in treating wounds, burns, and skin infections. In fact the use of honey accelerated the healing process when compared to other treatments, with no itching or skin irritations, pain, inflammation or foul odors. Instead, it promoted the growth of healthy new skin.

In his book *Folk Medicine*, Dr. Jarvis recommends chewing honeycomb cappings at least a month prior to hay fever season, to prevent hay fever starting.

A preparation using a mixture of dark honey, olive oil and beeswax containing pollen was trialed successfully in the Saudi Arabian medical center. It was used on 37 patients with fungal skin infections, and treated dermatitis and psoriasis (chronic skin disease).

Honey is an alkaline forming product within the body so helps to counteract the acidity which can promote rheumatism and arthritis, and will help in maintaining the body's health.

In 2004, a UK study used honey to treat 40 patients whose leg ulcers had been caused by poor circulation. Their ulcers had not responded to compression stockings (a product similar to flight socks). For the next 3 months, honey dressings were applied to the leg ulcers. As expected, the ulcers reduced in size and also made the associated pain more manageable.

Cancer Treatment

Interviewing cancer specialist Dr. Glenys Round confirmed that she had been using honey to successfully treat fungating wounds (an injury caused by the growth of a cancerous tumor through the skin), and the results had been excellent. She also had success in using honey to dress wounds and ulcers of patients suffering from radiation treatment.

Beekeepers who use propolis, honey cappings and other hive products in their diets are known to have a very low incidence of cancer. This is borne out by the longevity of the old Hunza beekeepers of Pakistan.

12

Royal Jelly

The activity of the hive can be somewhat confusing to many, so I am laying out this information as simply as possible, as the more you learn about these fascinating creatures, the more you realize how and why bees have established themselves and survived over millions of years.

One hive contains approximately 40,000 to 50,000 bees with one queen bee, and a ratio of at least 100 female (worker) bees for every individual male (drone) bee.

The queen bee is the lynch pin of the hive, or the 'Goddess.' I like to think of her as the mother of the hive. She lives for about two or three years, sometimes longer, and her role in life is to produce progeny for the hive by laying up to 1,500 to 2,000 eggs per day...she only leaves the hive once or twice in order to mate just the once in her lifetime.

Special cells in the hive are designated for raising queens. They are then fed royal jelly containing honey and pollen. Just a handful of queens live, and the first to hatch kills the remaining embryos so she can become the sovereign.

She is always surrounded by worker bees, feeding her royal jelly and looking after her social needs.

With the ingestion of this super supplement, she manages to outgrow the other bees—sometimes by as much as 60%. She is not easy to spot in the mass of bees within the hive and, as a result, the beekeeper will usually mark her abdomen with a spot of paint.

Drone Bees (male)

Drones are fertile male honey bees and are essential both for the survival of the bee colony, and also all future colonies. Their only role in the hive is to mate with the queen bee, to produce future progeny. They die soon after mating with the queen. Not a happy ending for them!

When a drone mates with a queen and releases his semen, it happens with such a force that his endophallus is torn from his abdomen, his abdomen rips open and he usually dies shortly after.

They can vary in size; they are smaller and stumpier than the queen bee, but larger than the female worker bee with a thicker abdomen. They help to keep the hive cool by flapping their wings.

What a relief, they don't have stingers!

Female Bees (workers)

Female bees outnumber the male bees by about 100:1, but they have many roles to carry out.

They perform all the work in the hive, looking after the cleaning, attending to the queen and, most importantly, feeding her 'royal jelly'. This is the only food that the queen consumes, hence her size being up to 60% larger than her companions.

Worker bees have **stingers** unlike the drones.

The females have varying tasks within the hive. Some act as guards at the entrance to the hive and keep all crawling insects at bay. If an insect manages to enter the portals of the hive they are duly dispatched and covered in propolis (i.e. mummified), in this way the hive is kept completely sterile and bacteria free.

The Value of Royal Jelly

Royal jelly is a creamy white substance which is fed to the queen bee by young female (worker) bees.

It is highly nutritious, and it is the only food that 'Her Majesty' consumes in her lifetime.

Royal jelly comprises:

Carbohydrates	18%
Lipids (organic fatty acid)	3 % to 6%
Water	50% to 60%
Mineral Salts	up to 2%
Proteins	18%

In her book *Royal jelly, Guide to Natures Richest Health Food,* Irene Stein describes how royal jelly helped to cure malnutrition in babies.

All of the babies gained weight and their immune systems were strengthened by the increase of red blood cells. With regular consumption, it was found that royal jelly improved the ability of the white blood cells to cleanse the body of bacteria and germs.

In 1998 Brazilian research proved that royal jelly had antiseptic and antifungal qualities which helped the skin to heal wounds more quickly, particularly in the case of eczema, dermatitis and impetigo (a highly infectious skin infection causing red sores in the mouth and nose area of children).

It has been found that in some cases impetigo bacteria had become resistant to antibiotic drugs.

Royal Jelly Therapy

Royal jelly has been observed to help regulate cholesterol levels, both HDL and LDL levels, as an aid to fertility and to improve blood pressure. According to the tabloid press, Princess Di in the UK used royal jelly as a food supplement to enhance her ability to produce royal heirs. History has proved that she was enormously successful.

A study by the University of Toronto found that mixing royal jelly with tumor cells before injecting them into laboratory mice proved eminently successful, whilst other mice injected with tumor cells died within two weeks.

A further successful study was carried out in Iraq by Ali e Al-Sanafi, Safaa A Mohssin, and others. 83 infertile men were given different amounts of royal jelly to increase their production of testosterone.

After 12 weeks the men who were given royal jelly and honey had improved sperm motility and higher testosterone levels. On the basis of the results, royal jelly was found to be safe and effective in the treatment of male infertility.

Chemotherapy research in 2016 found that royal jelly was able to protect patients from the usual negative effects of this drug.

Royal Jelly Dosage

Royal jelly can be eaten raw, but it is recommended that it is mixed with a little honey as on its own it is described as being rather bitter, and the aftertaste is unpleasant.

For optimum results, use 1/4-1/2 (1,250mg-2,500mg) per day, but make sure it is organically pure. Note: the properties of royal jelly are negated if heated. Fresh jelly should be kept in a refrigerator.

Royal jelly can be purchased in capsule form—in which case the manufacturer's advice should be followed.

If you are unsure about taking royal jelly, it would be wise to consult a medical practitioner before taking a daily supplement.

Weight Control

Another useful study carried out may prove helpful for diabetics who struggle with weight control. A 1,250mg dose of royal jelly was provided for diabetic patients, others were provided with a placebo.

After two months, patients were weighed and their daily diets recorded. The results were encouraging. Those taking the royal jelly lost 1.5kg (3lbs) of body weight, whereas the placebo group lost nothing and in fact actually increased their body weight.

Caution

As mentioned previously in the propolis section, a small percentage of the population can be allergic to bee products, whether honey, propolis, pollen, or royal jelly.

The allergic reaction in some cases can be obvious, causing skin rashes and in some cases breathing problems. To check any allergies, it is recommended to consume or try small quantities initially.

It has been recommended to avoid royal jelly if you have any of the following conditions/are taking any of the following medication:

- If you are estrogen receptive positive

- If you are taking cholesterol lowering medication

- If you are taking blood thinning drugs such as Warfarin or Xarelto/ Rivaroxaban.

If you are at all unsure, it would be advisable to always seek medical advice.

Finally, it's no wonder that pollen and royal jelly has developed such a reputation. Its ability to fight off infection, reduce inflammation, lower blood sugar levels (particularly useful for diabetics) and control weight mean it is a generally excellent health supplement.

13

Conclusion

For the past decade, hospitals worldwide have seen serious problems with bacterial resistance, with MRSA being just one, well-publicized example.

We face a worrying crisis of overuse and total dependence on chemical medicine, but to our credit we are all becoming aware of the benefits of natural products for combating diseases.

We have seen that propolis has proved it can alleviate many health problems with little or no side effects, and importantly it does not kill friendly bacteria, unlike antibiotics.

Propolis is not a cure-all solution for our ailments. A magic bullet does not exist. However, propolis could play an important role in the future, both in the home and in our hospitals, and has vast potential for human health.

I sincerely hope that my research has proved helpful in making you aware of a natural food supplement which could alleviate possible health problems now, and in the future.

Bee products are truly God's gift to us all. 'Bee Well' and remain in good health.

Your Questions Answered

FAQ about Propolis

Dosage

As propolis is classed as a food supplement and not a medicine there will not be dosage instructions on the packaging. I have indicated the dosage for the ailments listed above, using my own experiences and those of others.

The allergy specialist Dr. McEwen recommends a minimum dose of 1500mg. But Russian doctors who we know have decades more experience with the use of propolis are known to prescribe up to 9g-10g per day for some serious conditions.

In my experience, I have found it beneficial to take up to 3000mg per day for 2 weeks before a long flight, or when flu is prevalent and then taper down to my normal dose of 1g per day in capsule form, with no ill effects.

Allergies and Propolis?

As we now know, propolis is a natural food from the hive, and like all foods there is a possibility that a small number of people could have an allergic reaction to it, but toxicity is rare. It has been estimated that one person in 2000 can have a reaction to propolis and bee products, including beekeepers themselves. An allergic response can manifest as skin inflammation, redness and itchiness.

In fact, a paper published in 1967 by the Department of Dermatology in Edinburgh following up on the allergic reactions developed by beekeepers found that rashes were only prevalent during seasonal times when handling honeycombs and bees. They conducted case studies and patch tests to confirm this. In most cases, the condition was not evident during the winter months (when the beekeepers were not attending their hives).

Is it Safe for Children?

It is recommended NOT to give propolis to children, until they have blown out their first candle and then it should be given in a small dose to test for allergic response. In Murat's paper *Propolis the Eternal Natural Healer*, he recommends starting with half the adult dose, however taken, and then building it up gradually.

Is Propolis available for Vegetarians?

Capsules and tablets are available for vegetarians. Propolis liquids are recommended for a more immediate effective response, i.e. in the case of an asthma attack or severe infections.

Is Organic Propolis available?

Organic propolis is not readily available. As bees forage over an area of twelve square miles or so, it is not possible to guarantee that the bees forage within a completely organic environment which is free from all herbicides and pesticides.

Is it safe for animals?

Much of the research on the use of propolis in animals has been carried out in Eastern Europe and China. There have been some notable results, particularly in the treatment of cattle, pigs, poultry and sheep.

Many veterinarians are turning to natural products to treat our animals and pets including cattle, pigs, sheep and poultry, birds, cats, dogs, fish, rabbits and guinea pigs, racehorses, riding horses, and race hounds. Again, problems with antibiotics are driving this movement.

Veterinary practitioners are concerned both about the decreasing effectiveness of antibiotics and the public concerns about antibiotics in food; particularly with regard to how they may be increasing our own resistance to antibiotics.

Reports on the treatment of farm animals and pets with propolis have recorded some considerable success. It has been particularly useful in cattle production and treating skin disorders, infections and wounds.

James Fearnley's book *"Bee Propolis" Natural Healing from the Hive* gives more detail for those wishing further information. His company BeeVital is now producing a tincture of propolis preparation.

Is raw propolis available?

Raw propolis chips can be obtained from your local beekeeper. Just check first to make sure that it is clean and comes from an area which is environmentally friendly. Your local Beekeepers Association could help you here. The taste is not unpleasant, and when chewed has a slight numbing/anesthetic effect on the mouth. After a short time it changes to a consistency not unlike chewing gum.

This method of taking propolis is ideal for combating sore throats, gum disease, mouth ulcers, and even bad breath (halitosis).

Preparations of Propolis

Propolis tinctures are the easiest to make. This is the most common preparation and it has the maximum therapeutic effect.

Propolis chips can be broken into small pieces and stored in the freezer for a few days until they become brittle. Use a pestle and mortar or a coffee grinder to grind the chips.

The most commonly used solvent is alcohol. Food grade alcohol **must** be used, **not denatured alcohol** as this contains dangerous chemicals to prevent it being consumed.

Use about 40g of propolis powder and mix it with 100ml of 70% proof alcohol (or higher). Leave it in a warm dark place for 7 to 14 days, stirring daily. Use as little heat as possible as this can tend to damage the potency. Be aware that alcohol is highly flammable so keep it away from a direct flame source. For home use you can use vodka or gin as the solvent suspension.

After two weeks the solution should be filtered through fine muslin or coffee filters. Store the solution in a dark brown bottle in the refrigerator for a few days, and then filter again using as fine a filter as possible.

Store the liquid in the bottle away from direct sunlight. In this way it can be stored indefinitely.

Take a few drops daily, usually in a warm drink, to keep coughs and colds at bay. Or you can use it in your own honey to improve the potency of the product.

The tincture can of course be applied to cuts and grazes, infections and wounds.

Water Extract: Rather than using alcohol (which can sting slightly when used externally on open wounds), water can be used. Use 10g to 15g of propolis powder mixed with pure filtered water, after 24 hours, and shaking regularly, filter the solution as above.

The solution can be mixed with a small amount of mint, eucalyptus, lavender etc., and used as a nasal spray. Use a mechanical spray to treat burns and skin infections.

General Advice

The best way to take propolis is to try it gradually, only small amounts for the first few days. Afterwards, slowly increase the dosage assuming there were no side effects.

Also written by Colin Platt

- How to Cheat Colds and Flu
- The Back-Pain Survival Guide (released May/ June 2020)

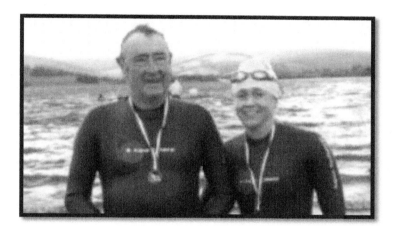

Taken after a 1-mile swim for charity with his daughter Pippa in 2013 when he was 75 years young!

Finally, I would appreciate it if you would review my book on Amazon, particularly if you believe we should be helping the world of the bees by providing nectar loving garden flowers and shrubs.

You can contact me at: colinp07@gmail.com

References

Dr. Ali F.M. Ain Shams University of Egypt Treatment of Infertility and mild endometriosis. October 2003.

Dr. Remy Chauvin 1980. Subject Propolis in the treatment of hay fever. Apiacta. 15/101/3

Osmanagic Izet 1976. Report on Influenza and its preventative properties Sarajevo.

Dr. Maximillian Kern, Ljubljana Clinic in Yugoslavia. Treatment of halitosis with propolis

Dr. Philip Wander 2005. 'Health from the Hive'. The applications of propolis in Dentistry.

Dr. Leonard McEwan 1996. The Allergy specialist. London. Treatments with propolis at his clinic.

James Fearnley LLB 2001 'Bee Propolis' Natural Healing from the Hive by Souvenir Press.

Dr. Bernard Jenson PhD. 1994. In his book 'Bee Well Bee Wise. Meeting with Russian beekeepers and their remarkable lifespan.

Dr. Philip Wander 1995. Paper. 'Taking the Sting out of Dentistry'

Murat, F. 1982. The uses of propolis. Propolis, 'The Eternal Natural Healer'.

Grange. J.M.and Davey, R.W. 1990. Journal of the Royal Society of Medicine. Positive results treating MRSA strains.

Hill R. 1977 'Propolis 'The Natural Antibiotic'. Thorsons Publishers Wellingborough England.

Choice Books and Resources

Bee Propolis. Natural Healing from the Hive. (2001) by James Fearnley. LLB. Souvenir Press.

Propolis the Natural Antibiotic (1977) by Ray Hill. Thorsons Publishers Ltd

Propolis Plus by Carlton Wade (1996) Wade & Keats Publishing Inc.

Users Guide to Propolis. Royal Jelly Honey and Bee Pollen by C.Leigh Broadhurst (2005) Basic Health Publications.

Bee Well Bee Wise (1994) by Bernard Jensen Ph.D. Publisher, Bernard Jenson.

Health and Healing with Bee Products (2002) by C Leigh Broadhurst, Alive Books.

A World Without Bees (2008) by Alison Benjamin and Brian McCallum, published by Guardian Books. A brilliant read 5* rating from me.

<u>**Association Addresses**</u>

American Apitherapy Society Inc.

www.apitherapy.org

British Beekeeping Association

www.bbka.org.uk

International Federation of Beekeepers Association

www.ibra.org.uk

Beekeeping Database

www.beedata.com

Magazine of American Beekeeping

www.beeculture.com

Apimondia, International Federation of Beekeepers Association

www.apimondia.org

<u>**Propolis Producing Companies**</u>

Natures Laboratory Ltd. (UK)

www.herbalapothecaryuk.com

www.beevitalpropolis.com

Comvita Ltd. (Bay of Plenty, New Zealand)

www.comvita.com

Stores in most major countries

The Propolis People (South Africa)

www.thepropolispeople.co.za

CC Pollen Co (Phoenix, Arizona)

www.ccpollen.com

Beehive Botanicals (Hayward, Wisconsin)

www.beehivebotanicals.com

Australian By Nature Pty Ltd (NSW)

www.australianbynature.com/au

Index

Printed in Great Britain
by Amazon

45257280R00068